5 MINUTES SOMATIC EXERCISES FOR BEGINNERS

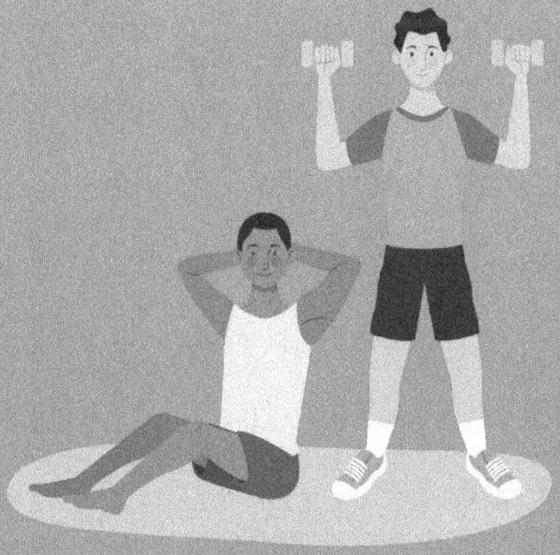

Quick and Easy Workouts with 4 Weeks Program for Novices to Revitalise the Body

Dr. Diane Reyes

Copyright © 2024 by Dr. Diane Reyes

Table of Contents

Introduction

It was just another hectic Monday morning and Sam's alarm blared, jolting him out of a deep sleep. As he shuffled to the shower, he could feel the tightness in his neck and shoulders from tossing and turning all night. "I really need to find time to relax," he muttered to himself.

The morning raced by in its usual frenzy of emails, meetings, and deadlines. By noon, Sam noticed his back starting to ache on top of the tense shoulders he woke up with. He popped a few painkillers to get through the day.

This scene is all too familiar for most of us living in the modern world. We wake up feeling exhausted no matter how long we slept. Our bodies ache from hours of sitting hunched over screens. Stress weighs on us mentally and physically.

As the day drags on, we reach for coffee, energy drinks, and pain medication just to cope with all the tension. But these are just quick fixes - not long-term solutions. What we're missing is real balance and body awareness.

The good news is you can reclaim your energy, health, and inner calm in as little as 5 minutes per day through the simple somatic exercises outlined in this book. Just taking a few mindful minutes to tune into your body can transform how you feel.

Within these pages, you'll discover easy somatic movements to release muscle tightness, improve your posture and alignment, breathe deeply, and quiet your mind. No special equipment or expensive classes needed.

The chapters offer modifications for every fitness level from beginner to advanced.

Follow the 5-minute routines in the book and soon you'll notice the aches fading away. Your sleep and concentration will improve. You'll feel less stressed and more energized. But the benefits go much deeper than physical relief - you'll build an invaluable mind-body connection that benefits every area of your life.

Why live with chronic pain and exhaustion when you can transform your well-being with just 5 minutes of practice a day? Apply these simple somatic techniques and move through your days with more ease, awareness, and inner calm. Your body and mind will thank you!

Getting Started with Somatic Exercises

Somatic exercises are a type of movement therapy that help improve mind-body awareness and physical functioning. As we become more sedentary and disconnected from our bodies in modern life, somatic practices can be beneficial for people of all ages and abilities. This article will provide an introduction to somatic movement and offer guidance on safe and effective somatic exercise.

What is Somatic Movement?

The term "somatic" comes from the Greek word "soma" meaning "body." Somatic practices emphasize tuning into the wisdom of the body and becoming more aware of subtle physical sensations.

Somatic movement is an umbrella term for therapeutic movement modalities that integrate body and mind through purposeful, attentive movement.

Some common somatic movement practices include the Alexander Technique, the Feldenkrais Method, Ideokinesis, and Authentic Movement. Somatic exercises are done slowly, gently and mindfully to foster neuromuscular coordination, postural alignment, strength, flexibility, and balance. The emphasis is on how the exercise feels internally, rather than achieving an external goal like building muscle mass.

Somatic movement teaches us to notice physical tension or disconnection and make small adjustments that help integrate the mental, emotional and physical aspects of being human.

Over time, increased somatic awareness can relieve chronic pain, improve posture and mobility, enhance self-image and body awareness, and reduce stress. Somatic practices bring us into the present moment through conscious embodiment.

Importance of Mind-Body Connection

Somatic exercises recognize the deep connections between mind and body. What we think and feel impacts our physical state, while our body's sensations and movements affect our thoughts and emotions. When we are stressed or disconnected from our body's needs, we are more likely to experience issues like neck and back pain, anxiety, and low energy.

Practicing somatic movements can help us identify unhealthy patterns like slouching, clenching, or shallow breathing. As we become more aware of our posture and movement habits, we can make small shifts to release tension, expand our breathing capacity, and move in an integrated, natural way.

These changes help calm the nervous system, improve coordination, and enhance mind-body wellness.

The mind-body integration cultivated in somatic movement is believed to tap into our body's innate wisdom to find balance, adaptability, and ease. Somatic practices help us get out of our head, reduce stressors on the body, and gain an inner sense of resilience. Connecting to the somatic experience has been shown to boost mood, self-awareness, and vitality.

Safety Precautions and Guidelines

It is important to keep some safety guidelines in mind when getting started with somatic exercises:

- Always listen to your body's signals and avoid pushing into pain. Move slowly and focus on control and coordination.

- Keep proper alignment to avoid undue strain. Engage core muscles, keep your spine elongated, and maintain balance between muscle groups.

- Stay present with your breath and avoid forcing your body into positions it finds difficult. Ease in and out of movements.

- Modify movements as needed based on your current physical condition. Don't compare yourself to others.

- Keep muscles warm to avoid pulls or strains. Wear comfortable clothing that permits free movement.

- Use caution if you have injuries, chronic pain, or postural issues. Consult a somatic practitioner if needed.

- Move slowly after sustaining an injury until you rebuild strength and flexibility.

- Ensure you have adequate space to move freely without obstruction. Use props like cushions as needed.

- Start with shorter practice times and gradually increase duration as your body adapts.

- Stay hydrated and listen if your body needs rest. Somatic exercises should leave you feeling integrated.

The key is tuning into your unique somatic experience without expectation or force. Increase awareness of alignment and sensation as you explore gentle movements at your own pace. With practice, somatic exercises can help you feel more embodied, energized, and relaxed.

The 5-Minute Routine Explained

Carving out even just 5 minutes a day for mindful movement can make a big difference in managing stress, easing body tension, and feeling more centered. The key is creating an environment conducive to a somatic practice and moving through a sequence of gentle warm-ups and breathing exercises tuned into your body. This simple morning routine can become an invaluable part of your self-care.

Setting the Right Environment

Set yourself up for success by creating a space that feels calming and removes distractions:

- Find a quiet room you won't be interrupted in. Silence your phone and close the door.

- Play some soft instrumental music if you find it centering. Avoid television or radio.

- Clear an open area you can move around in safely. Remove clutter and ensure good lighting.

- Use a yoga mat if you have one. Wear loose, breathable clothing.

- Have any props on hand you find supportive like cushions, blocks or a pillow.

- Allow yourself to mentally shift gears before starting. Sit quietly and become aware of your breath.

Tuning into your senses helps signal to your nervous system that you are entering a parasympathetic "rest and digest" state versus a fired-up "fight or flight" mode. Taking a few minutes at the start enables you to clear your mind, set intentions, and connect to the present moment.

Breathing Techniques for Somatic Exercises

Breathwork helps calm the mind and tune into the body before moving. Here are two easy 5-minute breathing exercises to try:

1. Square breathing - Inhale for 4 counts, hold for 4, exhale for 4, hold empty for 4. Repeat for 1-2 minutes.

2. Belly breathing - Place one hand on your chest, one on your belly. Inhale into your belly, feeling it expand. Exhale and feel it contract. Keep the chest still. Repeat for 2-3 minutes.

Consciously filling your lungs encourages relaxation and awareness. Spend at least a minute synchronizing your breath before starting to move. Deep abdominal breathing triggers the parasympathetic nervous system, providing a sense of calm.

Warm-Up Movements

After centering with your breath, warm up the body gently:

- Neck stretches - Drop your left ear to left shoulder. Inhale back to center, right ear to right shoulder. Repeat.

- Shoulder rolls - Lift and roll shoulders up and back in a circle. Reverse direction. Repeat 2-3 times.

- Torso twists - With feet planted, rotate your torso left, inhale back center, right side, exhale center. Repeat.

- Quad stretch - Use a wall for balance. Bend right knee, use left hand to pull right foot toward glutes until a stretch is felt. Hold 15 seconds, switch sides.

- Calf stretch - Step right leg back, left leg forward with knee slightly bent. Press into right heel until calf stretch is felt. Hold 15 sec, repeat on left.

- Cat-cow - On hands and knees, drop belly, look up as you inhale. Exhale to tuck tailbone under, arch back, look down. Repeat.

These are just some examples of mobilizing stretches and poses to wake the body up and lubricate the joints. Tune into areas of tightness and move slowly into them.

This short 5-minute sequence can be repeated daily to stimulate and integrate the body and mind. Listen to your body's needs in the moment - you may need more time warming up one day, and the next you may feel ready for deeper somatic movements. Stay adaptable and let your breath and awareness guide you.

Incorporating Somatic Exercises into Daily Life

The benefits of a regular somatic movement practice are immense, but it can be challenging to make time in a busy schedule. The key is starting small and integrating somatic exercises into your existing routines. With some creativity, you can bring mindful movement into your workday, morning ritual, and downtime.

Creating a Sustainable Routine

Begin by setting realistic goals for a home practice based on your current lifestyle and needs. Even 5-10 minutes 1-3 times per week can make a difference. Here are some tips:

- Schedule it like any other important activity and stick with it. Calendar reminders help.

- Try practicing first thing in the morning to start your day grounded and focused.

- Integrate it into your self-care routine, like after a shower or before bedtime.

- Follow audio or video guidance until you can remember flows. Apps and online resources offer variety.

- Start small, like holding a stretching posture for 5 breaths. Build up duration gradually.

- Be patient with yourself. It takes time for new habits to stick. Celebrate small wins.

Choose somatic exercises you enjoy and find relaxing, energizing or centering. Make sure to include standing, seated and lying down movements. Practice consistency for a few weeks until it becomes an intuitive part of your day.

Integrating Somatic Practices at Work

Look for opportunities to incorporate mindful movement into your work from home or office environment:

- Set reminders to pause and scan your body every hour. Release any tension.

- Do neck rolls or shoulder circles whenever you catch yourself slouching at your desk.

- Try walking meetings when possible to integrate movement with work.

- Take breaks to do a few sun salutations or stretches.

- Practice deep breathing techniques during stressful meetings or situations.

- Invest in a standing desk attachment to alternate sitting and standing.

- Take a longer mind-body break at lunch to reset. Find a quiet space.

- Organize group somatic exercises before meetings or yoga/meditation sessions after work.

- Replace your office chair with a stability ball to work your core.

Look for chances to decompress stress and re-energize through embodied awareness. Even small somatic breaks will boost productivity and wellbeing at work.

Quick Somatic Breaks Throughout the Day

Anytime your energy is flagging or you feel tense or distracted, take 1-2 minutes for a quick somatic reset:

- Shake out the body from head to toe. Release stuck energy.

- Roll your ankles, wrists, neck and shoulders.

- Stand in mountain pose with feet grounded and do 5 belly breaths.

- Slowly turn your head side to side, lowering ear to shoulder.

- Close your eyes and observe the weight and sensations in your body.

- Walk mindfully, paying attention to your footfalls and environment.

- Stretch your arms overhead, interlace your fingers, press palms up. Hold for 5 breaths.

- Do a standing forward fold, rag doll your upper body. Bend your knees.

- Child's pose on the floor. Rest your belly on thighs, reach arms forward.

Anytime you need to get out of your head, check in with your body. Let it move, breathe, stretch and restore as needed throughout your day. With regular practice, somatic exercise becomes an intuitive self-care ritual for relief and reconnection.

Troubleshooting and Common Mistakes

Somatic practices offer many benefits, but you want to ensure you are moving in a way that feels integrated and energizing for your body. It's normal to encounter some discomfort, limitations or missteps as you explore new movements. Being mindful and making adjustments will allow you to keep progressing safely.

Addressing Discomfort or Pain

Some somatic exercises may bring up discomfort or muscle soreness, especially if you are releasing long-held tension or have injuries. Here's how to respond:

- Back off or stop the exercise if sharp or shooting pain occurs. Consult a professional if it persists.

- For general soreness, ease into stretches gently until the discomfort dissipates. Don't force it.

- Remember to keep breathing deeply into problem areas to encourage relaxation and blood flow.

- Use props like blocks or cushions to modify movements to be more supported.

- Focus on areas of tightness or restriction to slowly unwind them through mindful repetition.

- Apply heat pads or take an Epsom salt bath to ease muscle pain after practice.

- Drink plenty of water before and after somatic movements to stay hydrated.

Discomfort is common as we build more awareness and release holding patterns. Be patient, move slowly, and talk to a somatic practitioner if concerns arise.

Adapting Exercises for Individual Needs

We all have unique bodies, mobility limitations and injuries to consider:

- If you have injuries or hypermobile joints, modify to keep them stable and supported.

- Avoid movements like intense backbends if you have spine issues. Opt for gentle twists.

- If knees or hips are sensitive, limit flexion and perform more standing postures.

- Those with balance issues can practice near a wall or chair to grip if needed.

- If wrists are weak, opt for fists or forearms instead of flat palms on the floor.

- If exercises require too much flexibility, bend knees, don't fold fully, or use props.

- Those with physical limitations can do adapted movements while seated.

Get creative about making exercises feel good in your body. Don't compare yourself to others.

Avoiding Overexertion

It's easy to get carried away and move too ambitiously when learning something new. Safeguard against overdoing it:

- Check in regularly about your energy levels and don't push through exhaustion.

- Build up slowly over weeks and months for greater benefits long-term.

- Hydrate well before and after practice and refuel with healthy foods.

- Avoid exercising on a full or empty stomach, which can lead to dizziness or nausea.

- Listen carefully to your body's signals of tension, fatigue or discomfort.

- Balance somatic exercises with plenty of rest to allow your body to integrate the movements.

- Reduce frequency if you experience headaches, stiffness or other concerning symptoms.

Somatic movements should leave you feeling enlivened and resilient. Go at your own pace and remember that small consistent efforts are best for sustainable change.

The key is tuning into your unique body with patience and compassion. Adjust as needed to find what works best for you. Over time, you will experience the transformative power of connecting to your body's innate wisdom through regular somatic practice.

Tracking Progress and Celebrating Success

When starting a new somatic movement practice, it can be challenging to see small improvements day-to-day. Tracking your progress and milestones is essential for staying motivated and realising the tangible benefits over time. Appreciating achievements along the way makes it a rewarding journey.

Importance of Tracking

Consistently tracking your somatic exercise routine and any shifts you observe will:

- Help quantify changes in flexibility, strength, balance, coordination, etc.

- Identify patterns in areas that are improving or need more focus.

- Keep you accountable to your goals and routine.

- Provide encouragement when progress feels slow.

- Prevent overdoing it or pushing your body too far.

- Allow you and your somatic teacher to customize your practice.

- Help set new goals as your abilities advance.

Try keeping a somatic journal to log practices, sensations, insights, poses mastered, adjustments needed, etc. Or use a tracking app to monitor progress. Checking in regularly boosts motivation.

Notable Changes and Improvements

Over weeks and months, you may start to notice:

- Increased flexibility, balance, and range of motion.

- Better mind-body awareness and ability to release tension.

- Improved posture, alignment, and ease of movement.

- Decreased muscle soreness or pain.

- Enhanced body awareness and connection.

- A calmer mind and ability to concentrate.

- More restful sleep and balanced energy levels.

- Greater self-confidence and body appreciation.

- Feeling revitalized and grounded.

- Quicker recovery from strain or injury.

Tracking helps identify subtle breakthroughs like holding a posture longer or deeper twist rotation. Each personal victory represents your body learning and integrating.

Building a Sustainable Somatic Exercise Habit

Use celebratory milestones as rewards and inspiration to deepen your practice:

- Note somatic exercise streaks in your calendar. Plan a nice treat after 30 days straight.

- Buy yourself new gear like yoga props or clothes when you achieve a goal.

- Share your progress and transformations with loved ones. Inspire each other.

- Gradually increase frequency and duration to keep challenging yourself.

- Join new classes or modalities when ready for fresh inspiration.

- Set new goals around strength, flexibility, balance, or mindfulness.

- Keep reminding yourself of all the mental and physical benefits.

Staying consistent is key - appreciate each new somatic habit formed. Tracking your journey makes it easier to notice and trust all the positive changes unfolding. Keep an open, patient mindset, take pride in your commitment, and let the results motivate you for the long haul.

Somatic Exercises for Relaxation

Neck and Shoulder Release

Instructions:

Sit or stand comfortably with your spine straight.

Inhale deeply, lifting your shoulders towards your ears.

Exhale slowly, allowing your shoulders to drop and relax.

Gently tilt your head to one side, feeling a stretch along the opposite side of your neck.

Hold for a deep breath in and out.

Repeat on the other side.

Continue this gentle side-to-side motion for 5 minutes, focusing on releasing tension with each breath.

Diaphragmatic Breathing

Instructions:

Find a tranquil space and sit or lie down comfortably.

Place one hand on your chest and the other on your abdomen.

Inhale deeply through your nose, allowing your abdomen to expand.

Exhale slowly through pursed lips, feeling your abdomen contract.

Focus on the rise and fall of your abdomen, keeping chest movement minimal.

Continue this diaphragmatic breathing for 5 minutes, allowing each breath to bring relaxation.

Seated Forward Bend

Instructions:

Get seated on the floor with your legs extended in front of you.

Inhale deeply, lengthening your spine.

Exhale as you hinge at your hips, reaching your hands towards your toes.

Relax your neck and shoulders.

Hold for a deep breath in and out.

Breathe in while gradually returning to an upright posture.

Repeat for 5 minutes, focusing on the gentle stretch and release in your lower back and hamstrings.

Mindful Body Scan

Instructions:

Recline on your back in a cozy position.

Shut your eyes and inhale deeply a few times to center yourself.

Start from your toes and mentally scan each part of your body.

As you scan, consciously release tension and let each body part relax.

Move slowly up through your legs, torso, arms, neck, and head.

Spend a few breaths on any areas of tension, allowing them to soften.

Continue the mindful body scan for 5 minutes, bringing awareness to relaxation.

Jaw and Facial Relaxation

Instructions:

Sit comfortably and close your eyes.

Inhale deeply through your nose.

Exhale slowly, letting your jaw relax and part slightly.

Massage your jaw with gentle circular motions using your fingertips.

Move on to your cheeks, temples, and forehead, applying light pressure.

Take deep breaths throughout, allowing facial muscles to release tension.

Continue for 5 minutes, focusing on the soothing sensation in your face.

Spinal Twist

Instructions:

Get Seated on the floor with your legs crossed.

Inhale deeply, lengthening your spine.

Exhale as you twist your torso to one side, placing one hand behind you and the other on your knee.

Hold for a deep breath in and out.

Breathe in, returning to the center, and repeat on the opposite side.

Continue this rhythmic spinal twist for 5 minutes, feeling the gentle release in your back.

Progressive Muscle Relaxation (PMR) for Arms

Instructions:

Sit comfortably and close your eyes.

Inhale deeply, clenching your fists.

Hold for a few seconds, then exhale as you release the tension.

Move to your forearms, biceps, and triceps, repeating the tense-and-release pattern.

Continue this progression through each muscle group in your arms.

Focus on the contrast between tension and relaxation.

Spend 5 minutes on this exercise, letting go of all tension in your arms.

Legs-Up-the-Wall Pose

Instructions:

Sit with one side against a wall.

Swing your legs up the wall as you lie back.

Adjust your position to bring your buttocks close to the wall.

Relax your arms by your sides with palms facing up.

Close your eyes and focus on your breath.

Hold the pose for 5 minutes, allowing the gentle inversion to bring relaxation to your legs and lower back.

Mindful Breathing with Body Scan

Instructions:

Sit comfortably with your back straight.

Close your eyes and take a few deep breaths.

Inhale deeply, feeling the breath travel through your nose and into your chest.

Exhale slowly, releasing tension from your chest down to your toes.

Mentally scan your body, acknowledging any areas of tension.

With each exhale, imagine releasing and softening those tense areas.

Continue this mindful breathing and body scan for 5 minutes, cultivating a sense of overall relaxation.

Butterfly Stretch

Instructions:

Sit on the floor with your feet together and knees bent outward.

Inhale deeply, lengthening your spine.

Exhale as you gently press your knees toward the floor.

Hold for a deep breath in and out.

Inhale as you release the pressure, allowing your knees to rise slightly.

Repeat this gentle pulsing motion for 5 minutes, feeling the stretch in your inner thighs and hips.

Somatic Exercises for Flexibility

Seated Spinal Twist

Instructions:

Get seated comfortably with your legs extended in front.

Breath in deeply, lengthening your spine.

Exhale as you twist your torso to one side, bringing one hand to the opposite knee.

Hold for a deep breath in and out.

Inhale back to the center and repeat on the other side.

Continue this rhythmic spinal twist for 5 minutes, feeling the gentle release in your spine.

Dynamic Arm Circles

Instructions:

Stand with feet shoulder-width apart.

Breathe in as you lift your arms to shoulder height.

Exhale as you rotate your arms in small circles, gradually increasing the size.

After a few circles, reverse the direction.

Continue this dynamic arm circle motion for 5 minutes, focusing on increasing shoulder flexibility.

Cat-Cow Stretch

Instructions:

Begin in a tabletop position on your hands and knees.

Inhale, arching your back and raising your head and tailbone toward the ceiling (Cow Pose). Exhale, rounding your back and tucking your chin to your chest (Cat Pose).

Flow between Cat and Cow poses, coordinating each movement with your breath.

Continue for 5 minutes, allowing the spine to flex and extend with each breath.

Dynamic Forward Fold

Instructions:

Stand with feet hip-width apart.

Inhale and reach your arms overhead.

Exhale as you hinge at your hips, folding forward and reaching towards the floor.

Inhale to a halfway lift, lengthening your spine.

Exhale back into the forward fold.

Continue this dynamic forward fold for 5 minutes, emphasising a fluid movement and gentle stretch in the hamstrings.

Ankle Rolls

Instructions:

Sit comfortably with your legs extended.

Lift one foot off the floor and rotate your ankle clockwise for a few circles.

Reverse the direction for a few circles.

Flex and point your foot, encouraging a full range of motion.

Repeat on the other foot.

Continue alternating ankle rolls for 5 minutes, focusing on mobility and flexibility in the ankles.

Lateral Side Stretch

Instructions:

Stand with feet wider than shoulder-width apart.

Inhale deeply, reaching one arm overhead.

Exhale as you lean to the side, creating a gentle stretch along your torso.

Hold for a deep breath in and out.

Inhale back to the center and repeat on the other side.

Continue this lateral side stretch for 5 minutes, promoting flexibility in the side body.

Seated Butterfly Stretch

Instructions:

Sit with the soles of your feet together, allowing your knees to fall outward.

Inhale deeply, lengthening your spine.

Exhale as you gently press your knees toward the floor.

Hold for a deep breath in and out.

Inhale as you release the pressure, allowing your knees to rise slightly.

Repeat this gentle pulsing motion for 5 minutes, feeling the stretch in your inner thighs and hips.

Dynamic Leg Swings

Instructions:

Stand next to a stable support (such as a wall or chair).

Swing one leg forward and backward in a controlled manner.

After a few swings, swing the leg side to side. Switch to the other leg and repeat.

Continue dynamic leg swings for 5 minutes, focusing on improving flexibility in the hip and thigh muscles.

Quadratus Lumborum Stretch

Instructions:

Sit on the floor with legs extended to one side.

Inhale as you reach your opposite arm overhead.

Exhale as you lean to the side, creating a stretch along your waist.

Hold for a deep breath in and out.

Inhale back to an upright position and repeat on the other side.

Continue this quadratus lumborum stretch for 5 minutes, promoting flexibility in the lower back.

Kneeling Hip Flexor Stretch

Instructions:

Kneel on one knee with the opposite foot in front, forming a 90-degree angle.

Inhale as you gently press your hips forward, feeling a stretch in the front of the hip.

Hold for a deep breath in and out.

Switch to the other leg and repeat.

Continue this kneeling hip flexor stretch for 5 minutes, focusing on opening up the hips.

Somatic Exercises for Stress Relief

Deep Belly Breathing

Instructions:

Sit or lie down comfortably.

Position one hand on your chest and the other on your abdomen.

Inhale deeply through your nostrils, enabling your abdomen to expand.

Exhale gradually through gently pursed lips, sensing the contraction of your abdomen.

Focus on the rise and fall of your abdomen for 5 minutes, calming the nervous system.

Gentle Neck and Shoulder Rolls

Instructions:

Sit or stand with a relaxed posture.

Inhale as you gently roll your shoulders backward.

Exhale as you roll them forward.

Add a slow neck roll in one direction, then reverse.

Repeat this sequence for 5 minutes, releasing tension from the neck and shoulders.

Grounding Body Scan Meditation

Instructions:

Get seated comfortably with your feet flat on the ground.

Get your eyes closed and take a few deep breaths.

Bring your attention to your feet, feeling the connection with the ground.

Gradually move your focus up through your body, acknowledging each body part.

Spend a few breaths on areas with tension, consciously letting go.

Continue this grounding body scan for 5 minutes, promoting relaxation and presence.

Somatic Self-Massage for Hands

Instructions:

Sit comfortably and bring your awareness to your hands.

Start by gently rubbing your palms together.

Massage each finger, paying attention to the joints and tips.

Rotate your wrists and massage the base of your thumbs.

Continue this self-massage for 5 minutes, promoting relaxation and soothing touch.

Somatic Release for Jaw Tension

Instructions:

Sit comfortably with a relaxed jaw.

Inhale deeply, allowing your jaw to open slightly.

Exhale and release any tension in your jaw.

Use your fingertips to massage your jaw joints with gentle circular motions.

Continue this somatic jaw release for 5 minutes, easing stress held in the facial muscles.

Mindful Walking Meditation

Instructions:

Find a quiet space for walking.

Begin walking in a slow pace, paying attention to each step.

Inhale as you lift your foot, exhale as you place it down.

Feel the connection between your feet and the ground.

Maintain a slow, deliberate pace for 5 minutes, focusing on the present moment.

Breath Awareness and Progressive Relaxation

Instructions:

Sit or lie down comfortably.

Get your eyes closed and take a few deep breaths.

Inhale, tensing your toes, then exhale, releasing the tension.

Move through each muscle group, tensing and releasing as you breathe.

Focus on the breath and the sensation of relaxation for 5 minutes, letting go of muscular tension.

Somatic Stretching for Back Relief

Instructions:

Sit on the floor with legs extended.

Inhale as you lengthen your spine.

Exhale and reach forward, allowing your back to gently curve.

Hold for a deep breath in and out.

Inhale as you return to an upright position.

Repeat for 5 minutes, focusing on the gentle stretch and release in your back.

Somatic Breath and Shoulder Release

Instructions:

Sit comfortably with relaxed shoulders.

Inhale deeply, lifting your shoulders towards your ears.

Exhale slowly, allowing your shoulders to drop and relax.

Rotate your shoulders backward and forward in a circular motion.

Continue this breath and shoulder release for 5 minutes, promoting relaxation in the upper body.

Guided Imagery and Relaxation

Instructions:

Find a quiet, comfortable space to sit or lie down.

Close your eyes and take a few deep breaths.

Imagine a peaceful place – it could be a beach, forest, or any calming environment.

Engage your senses in this mental imagery, focusing on the details.

Allow any stress or tension to melt away in this imagined serene setting for 5 minutes.

Somatic Exercises for Better Posture

Spinal Alignment Breathwork

Instructions:

Sit comfortably with your feet flat on the floor.

Inhale deeply, lengthening your spine and imagining a string pulling you upward.

Exhale slowly, engaging your core muscles to support your spine.

Continue this rhythmic breath for 5 minutes, focusing on maintaining a tall and aligned posture.

Shoulder Blade Squeezes

Instructions:

Sit or stand with your back straight.

Inhale as you squeeze your shoulder blades together.

Exhale and release, allowing your shoulders to naturally drop.

Repeat this shoulder blade squeeze for 5 minutes, emphasising the retraction and relaxation.

Chair Cat-Cow Stretch

Instructions:

Sit on a chair with your feet flat on the floor.

Inhale as you arch your back, pushing your chest forward (Cow position).

Exhale as you round your spine, tucking your chin to your chest (Cat position).

Flow between Cat and Cow positions for 5 minutes, promoting flexibility and awareness in your spine.

Desk Posture Reset

Instructions:

Sit at your desk with feet flat on the floor.

Inhale deeply, lengthening your spine.

Exhale as you draw your navel in towards your spine.

Lift your chest and roll your shoulders back.

Hold this upright, engaged posture for a deep breath in and out.

Repeat this desk posture reset for 5 minutes, preventing slouching and maintaining alignment.

Wall Angel Posture Exercise

Instructions:

Stand with your back against a wall.

Inhale as you raise your arms to shoulder height, pressing them against the wall.

Exhale as you slide your arms upward, forming a "Y" shape, and then back down.

Repeat this "angel" motion for 5 minutes, strengthening your upper back and improving shoulder alignment.

Pelvic Tilts for Lumbar Mobility

Instructions:

Sit or stand with a neutral spine.

Inhale as you tilt your pelvis forward, arching your lower back slightly.

Exhale as you tilt your pelvis backward, rounding your lower back.

Move through these pelvic tilts for 5 minutes, enhancing mobility in your lumbar spine.

Posture Check-In and Adjust

Instructions:

Set an alarm or reminder every hour.

Pause and assess your posture – check the alignment of your head, shoulders, and spine.

Make any necessary adjustments to maintain a neutral and supported posture.

Hold this improved posture for a minute, breathing deeply.

Repeat this posture check-in and adjustment throughout the day.

Seated Core Activation

Instructions:

Sit on a stable surface with your back straight.

Inhale deeply, engaging your core muscles by pulling your navel toward your spine.

Exhale slowly, maintaining this core engagement.

Continue this deep-breathing and core activation for 5 minutes, stabilizing your spine and supporting better posture.

Thoracic Extension Stretch

Instructions:

Sit or stand with a straight spine.

Interlace your fingers and place your hands behind your head.

Inhale as you lift your elbows, gently arching your upper back.

Exhale as you bring your elbows back down.

Repeat this thoracic extension stretch for 5 minutes, promoting flexibility in your upper back.

Somatic Awareness Walk

Instructions:

Stand tall with your shoulders relaxed.

Take a step forward, being mindful of your posture.

Focus on how your body feels with each step – from your head to your toes.

Engage your core and imagine a string pulling you upward.

Continue this somatic awareness walk for 5 minutes, maintaining a conscious and aligned posture.

Bonus: Somatic Diet Recipes

Breakfast Recipes

1. Berry and Yogurt Parfait

Ingredients:

1 cup of low-fat Greek yogurt

Half cup of mixed berries (strawberries, blueberries, raspberries)

2 tablespoons of honey

1/4 cup of granola

Instructions:

In a glass, layer Greek yogurt, mixed berries, and honey or a bowl.

Sprinkle granola on top.

Enjoy this nutritious and satisfying parfait.

2. Avocado and Spinach Breakfast Wrap

Ingredients:

1 whole-grain tortilla

1/2 ripe avocado, sliced

Handful of fresh spinach leaves

2 eggs, scrambled

Salt and pepper to taste

Instructions:

Place the whole-grain tortilla on a clean surface.

Layer avocado slices, fresh spinach leaves, and scrambled eggs.

Season with salt and pepper.

Roll up the tortilla and enjoy a protein-packed breakfast wrap.

3. Oatmeal with Almonds and Banana

Ingredients:

1/2 cup of rolled oats

1 cup of almond milk

1 banana, sliced

Handful of chopped almonds

1 teaspoon of honey (optional)

Instructions:

Cook rolled oats with almond milk according to package instructions.

Top with banana slices and chopped almonds.

Drizzle honey if desired.

A hearty and filling breakfast is ready.

Lunch Recipes

4. Quinoa and Chickpea Salad

Ingredients:

1 cup of cooked quinoa

1 cup of chickpeas, drained and rinsed

1 cucumber, diced

1 red bell pepper, chopped

Handful of fresh parsley, chopped

Juice of 1 lemon

Olive oil, salt, and pepper to taste

Instructions:

In a large bowl, combine cooked quinoa, chickpeas, cucumber, red bell pepper, and fresh parsley.

Drizzle using the lemon juice and olive oil, and season with salt and pepper.

Toss well and enjoy this refreshing and nutritious salad.

5. Grilled Chicken and Vegetable Wrap

Ingredients:

4 oz grilled chicken breast, sliced

1 whole-grain wrap

1/2 cup mixed grilled vegetables (zucchini, bell peppers, onions)

2 tablespoons of hummus

Fresh spinach leaves

Instructions:

Lay the whole-grain wrap on a clean surface.

Spread hummus on the wrap.

Add sliced grilled chicken, grilled vegetables, and fresh spinach.

Roll up the wrap and enjoy a protein-rich lunch.

Dinner Recipes

6. Baked Salmon with Asparagus

Ingredients:

6 oz salmon fillet

1 bunch of asparagus

1 lemon, sliced

1 tablespoon of olive oil

Salt, pepper, and dill to taste

Instructions:

Preheat the oven to 375°F (190°C).

On a baking sheet, place salmon and asparagus.

Drizzle with olive oil, season with salt, pepper, and dill.

Add lemon slices on top.

Bake for 20-25 minutes until salmon is cooked through and asparagus is tender.

7. Lentil and Vegetable Stir-Fry

Ingredients:

One cup of cooked green or brown lentils

1 cup of mixed stir-fry vegetables (bell peppers, broccoli, snap peas)

1/4 cup of low-sodium soy sauce

1 tablespoon of sesame oil

2 cloves of garlic, minced

1 teaspoon of ginger, grated

Instructions:

Heat sesame oil over moderate heat in a large pan.

Include the minced garlic and grated ginger, and sauté for two minutes.

Add mixed vegetables and cooked lentils, stir-fry for 5-7 minutes.

Pour soy sauce over the mixture and cook for an additional 2 minutes.

Smoothie Recipe

8. Green Protein Smoothie

Ingredients:

1 cup of spinach leaves

1/2 banana

1/2 cup of Greek yogurt

1 tablespoon of almond butter

1 cup of almond milk

Ice cubes (optional)

Instructions:

Blend spinach, banana, Greek yogurt, almond butter, and almond milk until smooth.

Add ice cubes if desired for a colder consistency.

Enjoy a protein-packed green smoothie to kickstart your day.

Juice Recipes

9. Citrus and Carrot Juice

Ingredients:

2 oranges, peeled and segmented

2 carrots, washed and chopped

1 lemon, peeled and sliced

1-inch piece of ginger

1/2 cup of water

Instructions:

Place oranges, carrots, lemon, ginger, and water in a juicer.

Process until you get a fresh and vibrant citrus and carrot juice.

10. Green Detox Juice

Ingredients:

1 cucumber, peeled and sliced

2 celery stalks

Handful of kale leaves

1 green apple, cored and sliced

1/2 lemon, peeled

Instructions:

Put cucumber, celery, kale, green apple, and lemon through a juicer.

Pour the green detox juice into a glass and enjoy the cleansing flavors.

SECTION III

Integrating Somatic Exercises into Your Routine

In this section, we provide tools to help you build a consistent somatic exercise routine into your daily life. Establishing regular somatic practice is key to experiencing the full benefits to body, mind and spirit.

We will outline a structured 4 week somatic workout plan you can follow, day-by-day. This removes the guesswork of what exercises to do each day.

Each day has two morning and two evening routines outlined, drawing from these somatic exercise categories.

In addition, we provide a journal template to record your experiences with each exercise session. Writing about your practice helps instill it as a habit and track your progress. Noticing improvements in how you feel gives motivational feedback.

Finally, we include a somatic exercise tracker chart you can use to check off each completed routine. This helps build accountability and consistency week-to-week in your practice. You can note any modifications or reflections after each session.

Our goal is to simplify starting and sticking with a regular somatic exercise routine. By following the structured 4 week plan, using the journal to record your journey, and checking off sessions in your tracker, you build sustainable somatic habits. In a month's time, you are likely to feel dramatic mind-body benefits that inspire you to continue the practices long-term.

4 WEEKS WORKOUT PLAN

Week 1

Day 1:

Morning: Deep Belly Breathing (Stress Relief - Exercise #1)

Evening: Seated Forward Bend (Flexibility - Exercise #3)

Day 2:

Morning: Dynamic Leg Swings (Flexibility - Exercise #8)

Evening: Mindful Body Scan (Stress Relief - Exercise #4)

Day 3:

Morning: Spinal Alignment Breathwork (Better Posture - Exercise #1)

Evening: Shoulder Blade Squeezes (Better Posture - Exercise #2)

Day 4:

Morning: Wall Angel Posture Exercise (Better Posture - Exercise #5)

Evening: Cat-Cow Stretch (Flexibility - Exercise #3)

Day 5:

Morning: Somatic Self-Massage for Hands (Stress Relief - Exercise #4)

Evening: Chair Cat-Cow Stretch (Better Posture - Exercise #3)

Day 6:

Morning: Grounding Body Scan Meditation (Stress Relief - Exercise #3)

Evening: Quadratus Lumborum Stretch (Flexibility - Exercise #9)

Day 7:

Morning: Breath Awareness and Progressive Relaxation (Stress Relief - Exercise #7)

Evening: Thoracic Extension Stretch (Better Posture - Exercise #9)

Week 2

Day 8:

Morning: Neck and Shoulder Release (Relaxation - Exercise #1)

Evening: Butterfly Stretch (Flexibility - Exercise #7)

Day 9:

Morning: Diaphragmatic Breathing (Relaxation - Exercise #2)

Evening: Dynamic Forward Fold (Flexibility - Exercise #4)

Day 10:

Morning: Seated Spinal Twist (Flexibility - Exercise #1)

Evening: Progressive Muscle Relaxation (PMR) for Arms (Stress Relief - Exercise #7)

Day 11:

Morning: Lateral Side Stretch (Flexibility - Exercise #6)

Evening: Legs-Up-the-Wall Pose (Relaxation - Exercise #8)

Day 12:

Morning: Mindful Breathing with Body Scan (Stress Relief - Exercise #9)

Evening: Kneeling Hip Flexor Stretch (Flexibility - Exercise #10)

Day 13:

Morning: Seated Butterfly Stretch (Flexibility - Exercise #7)

Evening: Mindful Walking Meditation (Stress Relief - Exercise #6)

Day 14:

Morning: Somatic Awareness Walk (Better Posture - Exercise #10)

Evening: Somatic Release for Jaw Tension (Stress Relief - Exercise #5)

Week 3

Day 15:

Morning: Chair Cat-Cow Stretch (Better Posture - Exercise #3)

Evening: Somatic Self-Massage for Hands (Stress Relief - Exercise #4)

Day 16:

Morning: Wall Angel Posture Exercise (Better Posture - Exercise #5)

Evening: Mindful Body Scan (Stress Relief - Exercise #4)

Day 17:

Morning: Grounding Body Scan Meditation (Stress Relief - Exercise #3)

Evening: Dynamic Leg Swings (Flexibility - Exercise #8)

Day 18:

Morning: Breath Awareness and Progressive Relaxation (Stress Relief - Exercise #7)

Evening: Seated Forward Bend (Flexibility - Exercise #3)

Day 19:

Morning: Shoulder Blade Squeezes (Better Posture - Exercise #2)

Evening: Quadratus Lumborum Stretch (Flexibility - Exercise #9)

Day 20:

Morning: Neck and Shoulder Release (Relaxation - Exercise #1)

Evening: Legs-Up-the-Wall Pose (Relaxation - Exercise #8)

Day 21:

Morning: Somatic Awareness Walk (Better Posture - Exercise #10)

Evening: Cat-Cow Stretch (Flexibility - Exercise #3)

Week 4

Day 22:

Morning: Diaphragmatic Breathing (Relaxation - Exercise #2)

Evening: Butterfly Stretch (Flexibility - Exercise #7)

Day 23:

Morning: Seated Spinal Twist (Flexibility - Exercise #1)

Evening: Progressive Muscle Relaxation (PMR) for Arms (Stress Relief - Exercise #7)

Day 24:

Morning: Lateral Side Stretch (Flexibility - Exercise #6)

Evening: Kneeling Hip Flexor Stretch (Flexibility - Exercise #10)

Day 25:

Morning: Mindful Walking Meditation (Stress Relief - Exercise #6)

Evening: Chair Cat-Cow Stretch (Better Posture - Exercise #3)

Day 26:

Morning: Wall Angel Posture Exercise (Better Posture - Exercise #5)

Evening: Mindful Body Scan (Stress Relief - Exercise #4)

Day 27:

Morning: Seated Butterfly Stretch (Flexibility - Exercise #7)

Evening: Legs-Up-the-Wall Pose (Relaxation - Exercise #8)

Day 28:

Morning: Somatic Awareness Walk (Better Posture - Exercise #10)
Evening: Somatic Release for Jaw Tension (Stress Relief - Exercise #5)

Journal and Tracker User Guide

Welcome to the Somatic Exercise Journal and Tracker, your dedicated space to record and reflect on your 4-week somatic movement journey. This journal will support you in building mind-body awareness and sticking with regular somatic practice.

Journal Structure

The somatic exercise journal is structured into 4 weekly workout trackers, with space each day to log your morning and evening practices. You can note the specific exercises, duration, and any helpful reflections. Tick each box as you complete sessions to see your progress stacking up.

After each week is a reflection note page. Here you can write about your experiences that week – challenges, benefits noticed, insights gained, positive changes emerging. Notice patterns over the month.

Additional tracker templates and reflection pages are provided to continue your somatic exercise routine beyond the 4 weeks if you desire. This journal can evolve with you.

Using the Journal

When using your somatic exercise journal:

- Record exercises done each day, even quick informal practices. Every mindful moment counts.

- Note details like duration, reps, modifications, intensity. Observe how these change.

- Reflect on sensations, breath, focus level. What did you learn about your body and mind?

- Tick each box with satisfaction as you persist through the 4 weeks. Let it be a visual mark of your dedication.

- In reflection pages, describe your inner experiences. Appreciate growth and insights gained.

- Re-read previous weeks to see your progression. Celebrate successes and growth.

This somatic journal is more than a log of exercises done. It is a space to deepen your inner awareness and relationship with your whole self – body, mind, spirit. Let it guide you in integrating the principles of somatics into your daily living.

Conclusion

The journey into somatic movement starts with a single mindful step - a commitment to reconnecting with your body's inner wisdom.

Through the gentle practices of somatic exercises, you learn to undo habitual tension, quiet your thinking mind, and tune into subtle physical sensations. Rather than forcing progress, you move with compassionate awareness.

An anti-inflammatory, whole foods diet provides nourishment to support your mind-body exploration. Conscious breathing techniques empower you to manage stress and access deeper states of calm.

Developing somatic competency is a process of unlearning – shedding patterns of exertion and disconnect. With patience and daily practice, you come home to yourself. Pain and anxiety yield to presence.

This book has outlined foundations and tools to guide you in awakening to the possibilities of the somatic path. Our hope is that the knowledge gained inspires you to continue your embodied evolution.

While the exercises herein are simple, their effects are profound. Movement becomes meditation when infused with mindful attention. You repattern the nervous system, resolve trauma in the tissues, and integrate all aspects of your being.

Trust in the innate inner wisdom of your body. Lean into sensorial experience. Let somatic exercises help you feel more at home, peaceful and empowered in your skin. Keep exploring this catalytic realm of healing connection.

The somatic journey is nothing short of a remembrance of your wholeness. May this book begin an expansive process of coming home to You.

BONUS: TRACKER AND JOURNAL

DAYS	EXERCISES	MARK

REFLECTION NOTE

REFLECTION NOTE

REFLECTION NOTE

REFLECTION NOTE

SOMATIC EXERCISE TRACKER

DAYS	EXERCISES	MARK

REFLECTION NOTE

REFLECTION NOTE

REFLECTION NOTE

REFLECTION NOTE

SOMATIC EXERCISE TRACKER

DAYS	EXERCISES	MARK

REFLECTION NOTE

REFLECTION NOTE

REFLECTION NOTE

REFLECTION NOTE

SOMATIC EXERCISE TRACKER

DAYS	EXERCISES	MARK

REFLECTION NOTE

REFLECTION NOTE

REFLECTION NOTE

REFLECTION NOTE

REFLECTION NOTE

REFLECTION NOTE

REFLECTION NOTE

REFLECTION NOTE

REFLECTION NOTE

REFLECTION NOTE

REFLECTION NOTE

REFLECTION NOTE